Wishes and Concerns of a Treated Asthma Patient

Due Consideration for Asthmatic People

By: James M. Lowrance © 2011

TABLE OF CONTENTS:

INTRODUCTION:

Many asthma patients (for which I am one), experience ongoing struggles, with frequent changes in their lung function. In addition to dealing with ongoing symptoms of breathing distress and worsening attacks of symptoms that can be severe or even life-threatening, we also have the added fear of not knowing where our asthmatic conditions will take us in the future, as we grow older. We may also at times, be unsure regarding our diagnoses, as far as to the type(s) of asthma we are suffering (i.e. asthma with elements of COPD, asthmatic Bronchitis, cardiac asthma, asthma of cystic fibrosis, etc…). Our doctors may in some cases, be non-compassionate and seemingly sloughing us off, rather than offering us the best possible treatment-options and reassurance that our diagnoses are definitive. These type issues are where the chapters of this book come from. I offer them as an asthma patient who experiences all of the fears and struggles I have just described. My expressed wishes and concerns that will follow are not to imply that I expect perfection in doctors or even in asthma treatments that continue to evolve into better ones, with each passing year.

Wishes and Concerns of a Treated Asthma Patient

You might say that I'm simply offering them (with some sincerely researched information sprinkled between them); to let my fellow asthma patients know that I understand their struggle.

For readers who are not asthma patients, I hope to convey to them an understanding of how our respiratory disorders can cause us genuine concerns and place a degree of limitations on our lives. Most of us know how to put on the brave face and to say the brave words from time to time and certainly we should remain as positive as we have the ability to be but as human beings, we all have our weak moments and frailties as well. While we are not seeking pity, we do simply want a reasonable degree of understanding, from our family, our friends and especially from our treating doctors. The American Lung Association so amply states it this way -- "When You Can't Breathe Nothing Else Matters".

It is my sincere hope that readers will find some nuggets of inspiration in the words I offer from the chapters of this book.

-*Jim Lowrance*

CHAPTER ONE:

My Personal Asthma Struggles: By Jim Lowrance

I also give my personal asthma story in my book titled: "What Do We Know about Asthma?" but in this account, I will mention a few additional aspects of it.

My asthma surfaced in me about 4 years ago but fairly mildly (it is now year 2011). It's currently moderate-persistent but fluctuates to a severe state depending on the time of year and can be mild or near-unnoticeable at times as well. I last had significant asthma symptoms in childhood but they resurfaced now in my late 40s after being practically non-existent and I believe acid reflux disease to be the direct cause of the relapse.

Over the past several years -- intermittently, I awakened from sleep choking on stomach acid and food particles, which left me wheezing. Over time, this apparently caused inflammation and possibly some damage to my lungs.

It also concerned me, that over time, I also developed orthopnea (harder to breath when flat on my back -- supine). Because this can be a heart enlargement symptom, I requested BNP blood tests from my doctor -- two of them over a year period and my results were very low on both results (the lower the better) and far-below the "100" high-normal cut-off that indicates mild heart failure if levels in the blood are at 100 and up to 300. Levels above 300 and up to 600 indicate moderate heart failure, while levels above 600 can mean severe cases. My two results were "4" and "16", so I was very happy to see that. For those of you readers, who might ever be concerned about heart failure, ask your doctor for the "BNP" blood test (B-type Natriuretic Peptide). It is 98% accurate in diagnosing heart failure (cardiac asthma) and the 2% questionable results, are likely those that are close to the high-normal cut-off range.

I also found through online search that orthopnea occurs in people with GERD and if you also have asthma, it makes sense that this can also worsen orthopnea. I also have Hashimoto's thyroiditis and hypothyroidism from it that is treated.

Recent studies have shown that people even with mild goiters can have a degree of orthopnea from them. On top of this, I'm moderately overweight and my midsection presses on my diaphragm when I lay flat on my back, so I actually have three contributors to my orthopnea, as related to my asthma (I do fine laying on my sides or stomach).

As the month of October approached in my mid US State, my asthma flared and I'm going through what actually feels like some bronchitis, this current fall season although I'm not producing a great deal of sputum (phlegm/mucous) and I am not experiencing fever. Mine instead feels like irritated lungs and as if I'm breathing-in cold air all the time. My doctor does currently have me on a 28 day round of Flovent Discus Inhaler. She actually should have prescribed it sooner, with all my asthma complaints at Dr. visits but I was previously only prescribed an Abuterol inhaler for the first several months.

I require the steroid type inhaler about once a year but have to specifically ask my doctor for it and I do use the Albuterol inhaler as much as needed.

Wishes and Concerns of a Treated Asthma Patient

Most patients with chronic persistent asthma, are on maintenance doses of inhaled steroids (low dose), year-round or at least for more than just a week or two within an entire year, as has been the case with me. I wish my doctor had better-treated my asthma, at its earlier onset and I might be seeing better days with it now and less or milder exacerbations of it (More about my doctor-dilemma, will be discussed in CHAPTER FOUR).

I will openly admit that as an asthma patient, even though never a smoker -- although my mom smoked when pregnant with me and I was around moderate second hand smoke till age 18, I still worry about the COPD possibility (some medical sources associate it with chronic GERD). This is likely a bit of hypochondria, which I think commonly, affects many asthma patients due to their concerning but very real symptoms, which in-turn can increase their worry and anxiety levels.

CHAPTER TWO:

Do Respiratory Crackles always Indicate Terminal Disease?

This article also comes from information I searched-out for a forum reply. I want to mention at the beginning of this one, that crackles heard in the lungs, also called "rales", can in some cases, indicate that a person is experienced symptoms of congestive heart failure or fibrosis of the lungs. In other cases, crackles can indicate bronchitis or pneumonia. It's also possible that some typical but severe cases of chronic asthma can cause occasional lung-crackles (i.e. asthmatic bronchitis). With this said, let's look at some information, following below, in which I point-out that other body organs can make sounds that may seem to be coming from the lungs. This is why true lung crackles/rales, should be diagnosed by a qualified medical doctor. Now to the information: ---

Quote: *"It is estimated that more than 75% of patients with asthma also experience frequent heartburn, a condition called gastroesophageal reflux disease (GERD)."* (from WebMD website)

I have some theories regarding crackling sounds that may come from the lungs in typical asthma or that might "seem" to be coming from the lungs. The first theory (I'm pretty sure about this), is in regard to me personally.

I feel that when I use my albuterol inhaler, especially if I use it 2 or 3 times in one day (very seldom), I may hear a few crackles at night in bed. I feel this is due to the medication loosening any mucous trapped in constricted bronchi-passages. Keep in mind that some asthma patients may have a great deal of anxiety after seeing a medical web page stating that crackles can mean COPD, Heart Failure or Pulmonary Fibrosis and understandably so.

This can make the frustration of not knowing if one of these things might be the case with them, when medical site pages contradict each other. Do they contract at times in a diametrically opposed fashion? Yes they do and I'm talking about sites that have articles on them by medical doctors. With this said, I greatly appreciate these sources and I have benefited from them many times.

Examples:

Some medical information sites state that pulmonary fibrosis is indicated if crackles occur early during inspiration (inhaling) and others state that it is indicated when they occur late during inspiration.

One medical site I read on (a U.S. Gov one), states that pulmonary fibrosis does not present the same as obstructive lung diseases do, such as asthma and other types of COPD (i.e. they specifically noted that they don't wheeze, don't have sputum producing coughs and their condition is not 'episodic'). During the same search I was doing, using same key words, I read an article by a licensed nurse practitioner, stating that patients with pulmonary fibrosis can feel well at times, only to experience episodes of worsening and that they experience wheezing (hence we have opposing opinions being expressed).

I read on other sites stating that crackles (rales) can only be heard with stethoscope; with others stating that they can often be heard without the use of one.

Similarly, some state that pulmonary fibrosis is detected by a typical chest xray (radiograph), in-fact some specifically stated that it appears on 85% to 90% of frontal chest xrays (but further confirmed by HRCT), while at least one other site stated that it "seldom" appears on chest xrays and only appears on HRCT. I've seen YouTube videos and I know for a fact that it definitely can appear on a typical chest xray, especially past the early stages, when definitive symptoms are occurring.

I'm not knocking medical info-sites - thank God for them but... it amazes me at how even the most reputable ones can contradict each other with information of this type.

Now to my theories about what might be heard as crackles, seemingly originating from the lungs: ---

In some cases, it is mucous or even saliva at the back of the throat or in the upper airways. Other times, it could be small crackling sounds coming from the spine, the sinuses or the esophagus. These can very much sound like they occur pulmonary because these same body areas are moved-around by expansion of the lungs.

I feel that true crackles will be extremely obvious (some medical sites have short audios of them you can play and they are unmistakable and come in strings of many, rather than a couple of snaps, crackles or pops here and there).

Not only is gastroesophageal reflux disease common in asthma patients (something I have experienced for years) but Laryngopharyngeal Reflux (LPR) is as well and they are two distinct disorders, the later often occurring together with GERD and can result in constriction of the larynx and or trachea over time (stricture). GERD can also cause esophageal damage and remodeling of it, called "Barretts Esophagus". All of these can result in increased throat sounds and in my opinion can easily be mistaken by the person breathing, as lung sounds.

I also find it suspicious that me and other asthma patients who have posted about crackles, seem to hear them when they are lying down at night but not when they are standing or sitting, even in a very quiet environment (I have tried this and the crackles disappear when not supine).

Wishes and Concerns of a Treated Asthma Patient

Just a quick mention that I have had two chest xrays in a year and a half period and my heart is normal size with no pleural effusions inside or surrounding my heart or lungs. The two BNP blood tests I had done (98% accurate in ruling out enlarged heart) were very low readings (low means no heart-stretching).

While I will be going to a pulmonologist in the near future, I truly believe my own intermittent crackles to be esophagus and possibly larynx or trachea related at least part of the time and the remainder of the time, might be from episodes of asthmatic bronchitis. I will also be seeing a gastroenterologist, due to concern that I likely have some upper digestive problems that are also contributing to my asthma.

CHAPTER THREE:

Naturally Treating Gastroesophageal and Laryngopharyngeal Reflux - Aggravators of Asthma

Subtitle: Lifestyle Changes and Natural Remedies for GERD

I suffer from the most common respiratory ailment that exists, being that of asthma, as previously mentioned.

My Childhood Asthma

My asthmatic symptoms actually first manifested when I was a child but from about my teen years forward, I saw relief from the flares of distressed breathing, which in my case, seemed to be triggered by being outside in very cold temperatures and after hard physical activity. My asthma actually resolved and my symptoms did not reappear for several decades. My immune system seemed to be compromised early in life however, with my experiencing more colds and viruses than did my siblings.

This included mononucleosis and afterward, my development of adult autoimmune hypothyroidism, at about age-40.

Conventional Treatments I Used for Adult Onset Asthma caused by GERD

The term "GERD" is simply an abbreviation for Gastroesophageal Reflux Disease and medical sources state that approximately 75% of asthma sufferers also experience chronic GERD. As I reached my mid-forties, I began seeing a return of asthma symptoms, which they actually refer to as "adult onset asthma" and this time, I believe mine to have developed from many years of chronic acid reflux disease.

I actually began taking prescription acid blocking medications, in my late 20s but as time went by, these drugs became available, over-the-counter. Some of the brands I took at different points, to control the acid that was coming from my stomach and up into my esophagus, that are also referred to as "proton pump inhibitors", included Zantac, Prilosec, Pepsid and Prevacid.

The Possible Long-term Side Effects of Acid-Reducer Medications

According to some medical sources, taking acid reducer drugs for more than a few weeks at a time can actually cause malabsorption of essential nutrients with long-term use, including causing low potassium (a recent finding in my own blood test results). Medical sources also state that drugs of this type can increase the risk for pneumonia in susceptible individuals (i.e. older adults and people with compromised immune systems). This is why I feel it is so important that we, who have respiratory illnesses, have natural alternatives and lifestyle practices that we can rely on, to help us deal with symptoms and to avoid the possible complications of extended acid blocker drug use.

Natural and Lifestyle Methods for Controlling GERD

One very important set of lifestyle practices to help with asthma when the suspected cause is acid reflux disease is to avoid spicy foods or beverages and those that are high in refined sugars or that contain caffeine, alcohol or other stimulants.

These type foods and beverages can cause a sudden increase in stomach acid production. Some GERD sufferers actually have "low stomach acid" but it can be the wide fluctuations in digestive juices that cause it to rise into the esophagus. The other problem is the refluxing action which causes increased esophageal contractions that push not only the stomach acid upward but also foods that have been eaten. Not eating too-close to bedtime can help with this as well, as can elevating the head of your bed by about six inches, using books or bricks under the legs of the head post. This prevents any acid from rising into the throat, which in-turn prevents aspiration of it into the lungs, which can result in asthma symptoms.

Herbs and natural products that have been reported to help with indigestion and GERD symptoms in general include the following.

* Apple cider vinegar
* Barley grass
* Bladderwrack
* Cabbage juice

19

Taking Necessary Precautions with Herbals

These herbs and natural products can be found at
health food stores and the containers they come
in, will state the recommended amounts that one
should take or when buying the products, one can
inquire about recommended dosing with store
representatives. Doing an online search, using the
name of the herbal being considered can yield this
information as well. This will safeguard against
the possibility of taking either inadequate
amounts of the supplements or taking higher
amounts than is recommended. I would also
suggest reporting use of any herbal remedies to
your MD, as a precaution, to make sure he or she
doesn't feel that they will not contraindicate with
any treatments you might already be taking (cause
adverse effects when combined with prescribed
pharmaceuticals).

Sources:

U.S. National Institutes of Health ("Uses of
proton pump inhibitors and serum potassium
levels"):
LINK:
http://www.ncbi.nlm.nih.gov/pubmed/19557730

Wishes and Concerns of a Treated Asthma Patient

U.S. National Institutes of Health ("Use of proton pump inhibitors and H2 blockers and risk of pneumonia in older adults")
LINK:
http://www.ncbi.nlm.nih.gov/pubmed/20623507

Laryngopharyngeal Reflux: Another Trigger for Asthma

Some medical sources do say that the association of GERD as a "cause" of asthma has not been clearly established. Others say it has been well confirmed -- this in-fact is where frustration can happen when people with health conditions do searches regarding their symptoms.

In some cases people actually come away from a search with some "cyberchondira" -- a very real anxiety disorder that has actually had research studies done on it.

I read an article recently for example, in which an MD who wrote a research paper, states that "frequent throat clearing" can be a symptom of idiopathic pulmonary fibrosis (an irreversible, terminal lung disease).

While I could never dream of having the knowledge an MD has, I feel he should have qualified that statement by adding that it's also a common symptom in asthmatics, in people with GERD and in those with post nasal drip and allergies (not for the sake of other medical people who understand the specific angle he was writing from but for non-pro medical patients who hugely outnumber doctors reading on the world wide web).

Also: Some patients resort to online search because their doctors do not take time to adequately inform them about their health disorders, due to time constraints.

This being said, it is important for us to be careful what we share through articles or on fellow patient forums and message boards but I also believe information can benefit a great deal, along with personal experience, if we do it in a balanced way, comparing several reputable sources together if possible.

I would like to add a quote that also associates the condition called Laryngopharyngeal reflux (LPR) to asthma.

LPR is A condition distinct from GERD but that often occurs together with it and following is a quote from a statement by the Journal of Asthma:

"Symptoms of LPR are often noted only as throat irritation similar to that caused by post-nasal mucous drainage. This may result in frequent throat clearing, throat fullness or pain, cough, hoarseness or problems during inspiration called "stridor." In addition
to causing stridor, LPR can also trigger asthma in asthmatics ...

This study suggested that 3/4th of all patients with mild to moderate asthma may have LPR (and most persons are usually unaware of it). LPR should be suspected in anyone with poorly controlled asthma and this study demonstrated that medical treatment could significantly improve asthma symptoms." (Publication: Journal of Asthma, 43; 539-42, 2006)

(NOTE: "Stridor" is defined by medical sources as abnormal sounds heard on inhale/inspiration.)

CHAPTER FOUR:

Doctors who Offer Inadequate Asthma Treatment

This may appear to be a somewhat off-beat subject for a chapter on the subject of asthma however; I feel it is an important one. It is by no-means meant as an attack against doctors generally. The medical profession is one I have great respect for and a good physician is one of the most valuable things one can find in life but at the same time, health disorder patients should know how to recognize insufficient health care from doctors they may be seeing. This can help them to avoid an unnecessary worsening of their health disorder and to find a good doctor who will treat them as optimally as possible, so that they can experience a better quality of life.

I will be citing my own experiences with a previous doctor following below, which provides examples of what asthma patients should look for that, might prompt them to seek a new doctor for their asthma treatment. I will also add that asthma specializing doctors are certainly the best option.

This of course includes pulmonologists (doctors of pulmonology) however; some asthma patients are simply unable financially to secure care from one. When this is the case, a qualified MD becomes the consideration.

I'm currently having a severe struggle with my asthma as previously mentioned (October of 2011) and I'm convinced I have upper airway problems of some type that are not sinus related (I believe much of it is upper-digestive and aggravating my asthma). I'll only be able to be diagnosed as to cause, once I can see a Doctor who knows what they are doing. I just canceled my previous Doctor and I will not attend more office visits due to my having to literally pull information out of her. She actually offered me a spirometry test a year and a half ago (a lung peak flow volume measurement that's more detailed than that you can obtain with a simple home peak flow meter) and despite both my wife and I reminding her about it, she continued to not bring the machine into her office to perform the test (almost certainly because of time constraints and being overbooked with office visits). Needless to say, this is why I am scouting for a new doctor now.

Wishes and Concerns of a Treated Asthma Patient

I will only add, to give further example of why I feel I was not getting proper care from this doctor; that I called her office about having severe, hard-to-control asthma symptoms that manifested like bronchitis. This, in spite of using a glucocorticoid inhaler that I previously had to ask her for -- a "Flovent Discus", which should have been offered or a similar medication, rather than my having to suggest it. Her reply was to say that I should rinse my mouth after each inhaled dose of the glucocorticoid (?)!

The reason this reply seemed like a slough-off to me is due to the fact that I did not say that I had problems in my mouth (oral thrush can occur if you fail to rinse your mouth when using Flovent -- which I was not failing to do).

I was very specific that my lungs were highly irritated and that my asthma was flaring severely and while prescription inhaled medications can potentially cause this as a side-effect, my doctor should have been willing to communicate with me regarding this and to rule-out other possibilities such as bronchitis, needing antibiotics.

I Know for a fact that there are good doctors available and I'm hoping to find one to replace my previous one, who appears to be experiencing burn-out, which seems obvious due to her lack of interest and compassion for patients (my mention of this to one of her nurses, was met by strong denial and the doctor would almost certainly deny this as well).

I would recommend this same action to patients who also believe their doctor is not providing them proper treatment for an asthmatic condition or other serious health disorder because bad medical treatment is the third leading cause of death in the US and patients must take a stand in helping to see changes in this problem over time. Even medical research groups are reporting that the "doctor burn-out problem" is worsening and causing increasingly inadequate health care for medical patients.

I also had childhood asthma and was around second-hand smoke until about age 18 or 19, as previously mentioned but only moderately and with 30 years of not being around it, my lungs should have recovered from the effects.

My asthma didn't recur until just a few years ago -- mildly at first. In spite of my mentioning atypical symptoms to my ex-doctor (i.e. occasional crackle sounds or what might be called clicks and wheeze on the inhale - mostly at night), my doctor would not offer me any input and simply prescribed an Abuterol rescue inhaler. She only prescribed me the medication inhalers, like the one I'm on now (Flovent Discus 250mg – for long-term asthma control), when I called at certain points of the year to complain that my asthma was flaring severely. In all likelihood, my asthma has worsened because I should have been on a medicated/steroid inhalant sooner. I also believe my crackle sounds when breathing which are intermittent and only occur on-occasion at night in bed, are due to my GERD (acid reflux -- mucous and irritation in throat). My doctor, who I just left, has also been aware of this problem for about two years and though she gave me samples of a prescription acid reducer drug (at my request), she never suggested that I should have an endoscope or similar evaluation done on my esophagus. Properly fixing a GERD problem, can significantly improve asthma conditions, according to medical information websites.

Wishes and Concerns of a Treated Asthma Patient

Anyway, that's how it goes in this sometimes inconsiderate world and I've read the testimonials of many other patients who've suffered from inadequate asthma treatment from their doctors as well. I honestly believe that while pulmonary specialists are certainly best, regular MDs and GPs should know enough about asthma -- one of the most highly experienced diseases that exists (affecting from 16 to 18 million adults in the U.S.), to know when proper meds should be started as treatment for it. If they feel cases are beyond their scope, they should give patients referrals to pulmonologists… and that's the obvious answer, to a potentially very serious problem in my opinion.

CHAPTER FIVE:

More Thoughts Regarding Cardiac Asthma

I've never had heart problems, am a non-smoker and in the year-2001 I had a normal stress test - EKG. My blood pressure is usually normal but at times borderline-high. I also do not experience any swelling in my feet or ankles or what they call pitting edema, which is characteristic of an enlarged heart, also called "heart failure".

I've never actually experienced fluid build-up in my lungs, which can also be a symptom of heart failure - mine is more-so small amounts of phlegm I get rid-of by simply clearing my throat (thick, sticky secretions, rather than a thin fluid type). I do wheeze, especially at night and feel the sensation of tight breathing passages.

I'm age-49, this year of 2012 but my asthma has been developing for years and just reached need for mild treatment last year. I did have asthma as a child as well but the condition left me completely for a number of years (at least 30 years) – or at least it seemed-to subside for that period of time.

Wishes and Concerns of a Treated Asthma Patient

I'm treated for hypothyroidism which was found at the mild stage when I was age-40, caused by Hashimoto's thyroiditis. I was also found to be vitamin D deficient in more recent years (flagged low) and I'm being treated for that and for vitamin E deficiency, plus for a milder B12 insufficiency (low-normal findings of this one, via blood tests). I've had Chronic Fatigue Syndrome symptoms for about 7 years - not corrected with optimal thyroid hormone dosing, so my immune system is apparently a bit compromised.

My suspicion is that some people with asthma do feel more breathing difficulty in the supine - flat on the back position but very few sources out there mention it. In my case, lying on my sides or stomach doesn't labor my breathing but on my back, my extra weight from being a bit obese in the mid-section (230lb at 6ft tall) may be pressing-down on my already constricted bronchial passages, when I lay on my back, placing more pressure on my diaphragms.

I searched and found very little in regard to the common garden variety of asthma and breathing difficulty in the supine position.

The source that did give most detail on it was this one -- WrongDiagnosis.com/Health Grades, Inc. -- http://www.rightdiagnosis.com/symptoms/orthopnea/common.htm, which states :

"Causes of Orthopnea that are "very common" - The following causes of Orthopnea are diseases or medical conditions that affect more than 10 million people in the USA:

* Asthma
* Chronic obstructive pulmonary disease
* Sleep apnea
* Panic attacks

Causes of Orthopnea that are "common" - The following causes of Orthopnea are diseases or conditions that affect more than 1 million people in the USA:

* Congenital heart diseases
* Congestive heart failure
* Emphysema
* Gastroesophageal reflux disease
* Myocardial infarction"

If you'll notice, the sources that are "very common" include asthma and the sources that are "common" include congestive heart failure.

What is also interesting is that acid reflux can be a cause of orthopnea. Each of the conditions listed in the very common category affect over 10-million people each, while the ones in the common category each affect about 1-million people each.

I also found a source that stating that orthopnea indicates heart failure in almost 95% of cases but this had to be an error because when you look at the lists of causes I referred to, or even just comparing regular asthma to the heart-related, this cannot possibly have been an accurate statement. I found the reference on two sources but they should be cautious about stating that type of statistic in my opinion. It could cause people with typical asthma to become unjustly fearful (cyberchondria) if they experience a degree of orthopnea. I didn't find the source until after I had my own testing done to rule out heart enlargement, in my own case.

I could still see that such a statistic should be well-confirmed and not just added as a sentence in an article about orthopnea.

What makes the claim that "95%" of people with orthopnea have heart failure, literally impossible to be true, is the huge difference in numbers of people with typical versus cardiac asthma. Common sense says this particular statement is lacking proper perspective (respectfully).

I believe they are actually meaning to convey in that statement, that 95% of diagnosed cases of CHF, presented with orthopnea as a symptom. That makes a lot more sense and very likely what they actually intended by it.

As far as anxiety triggering asthma attacks and potentially causing or contributing to orthopnea, this is mentioned on most detailed medical sources about asthma (not just anxiety but stress and even a joyful emotion can do so). Some also mention laughter as a trigger for attacks in some people. Also the reverse is true - if a person has an asthma attack, it can trigger panic symptoms.

This is basically what I was experiencing at times when I felt chest-tightness, when my asthma began to fully manifest a few years ago. I feel it is obvious that anxiety and asthma are highly associated with each other.

I had my chest xray done approximately 18 months ago and it was reviewed by the usual two MDs and my heart was found to be normal size and no signs of cardiopulmonary problems were found. This was also true of a second, more recent chest xray I had ordered.

What I was most happy to get back, was my result on my BNP blood test (B-Type Naturietic Peptides) test that I mentioned earlier. It is a fairly newly developed diagnostic test to detect heart failure and my result came back at "4". The lower the reading, the better an indicator of good heart functions.

It bears repeating, that the normal range is <100, so if you have a result of 100 or more on the test, it can indicate developing heart failure. One medical source I went-to, a cardiology college stated that a reading at "300" indicates mild heart failure.

At "600" it indicates moderate and at "900" indicates severe. It is a hormone that comes from the heart and floods the bloodstream, after it enlarges and there is stretching of the heart-muscle. Once this occurs the enlargement continues until it is treated and one of the treatment goals is to reduce the BNP level because the lower they can get it, the better the prognosis for patients. Most cases of the condition are in elderly people but it can occur in younger individuals when heart defects or injuries are present as well.

I also had the test done because I have a small band of swelling around my ankles at times but isn't in my feet or legs - it's just a two inch wide area of thicker area that appears at times and then goes away but I suspect arthritis because my feet and ankles hurt when I walk significant distances. Actually the type swelling heart failure patients experience is called "pitting edema" which means an indentation is left in the skin when pressed-down firmly for 30 seconds and this will most-often be in the feet and lower legs. My lower-body tissue never pits when I test for this with fingertip pressure.

Yet a third reason I had the tests done that I have described, was due to my occasional spells of frequent urination which can mean heart failure as well but apparently I have other things going on, causing some of these things. I had kidney disease and diabetes ruled-out through blood testing as well. My creatinine and BUN kidney tests were normal and both my blood and urine glucose readings were as well. So I'll simply need to keep an eye on these symptoms to see if they become significant at any point or if any changes occur in them. I actually feel they may be related to my thyroid disease - Hashimoto's thyroiditis/hypothyroidism which is treated well but this doesn't mean I won't see signs of thyroid disease in my body. The BNP blood test I also mentioned getting -- which came back negative for heart enlargement, according to the top online medical sources, is highly sensitive and accurate, should one want to rule-out heart involvement in their asthma. The test of course doesn't rule out all heart problems such as blockage or valve problems (this requires stress tests, other blood evaluations and echo cardiogram imaging) but it does detect or rule out active heart failure at the time of lab analysis.

CHAPTER SIX:

Asthmatic Bronchitis: Could Some of Us Have It?

I posted the information that follows below, on an asthma patient support forum, some time ago and I wanted to include that information as a chapter in this book. ---

"Fellow Asthma patients,

I ran across information on a condition called "asthmatic bronchitis" that I found very interesting and I believe this to be very likely the type of asthma flares I sometimes experience. The reason I say this is because I actually mentioned to my wife, that my persistent asthma flares (the more noticeable long-term ones, occurring only about once-yearly for the past two years) seem a great deal like bronchitis but without fever or huge amounts of sputum being coughed up (Also: I've never been a habitual smoker). Still the mucous/phlegm I do have coming up, is constant during these flares and requires me chronic throat-clearing.

Wishes and Concerns of a Treated Asthma Patient

I do have some coughing spells (mostly at might), which triggers more of the mucous, to come up into my throat from my lungs but I cough less than most asthmatics do.

I know the passages of my lungs are clogged during these flares and that they are inflamed and constricted as with asthma but mine have a tendency to not release the mucous, so that I can clear it out. A medicine like Mucinex would likely help me at these times when I can't seem to clear the obstructed passages, at least for a period of time (I know it will return due to the nature of asthma).

I do know that the feeling of congestion in my chest can be a very uncomfortable one, especially because it causes a feeling like I can't fully take-in a breath or sometimes fully expel one and as-if my intake of oxygen, isn't hitting the mark as it should (not being absorbed properly). I also feel an irritation in my lungs at these times, as if they actually hurt just a bit – like when you have a cold that goes to your chest and I get an instant urge to cough if I take-in a deep breath during these flares.

Anyway, my present bronchitis type manifestation of my asthma came this year, when the weather changed in my area, to colder temperatures. The sources I read that listed triggers for asthmatic bronchitis, included "weather changes" and also "GERD" (Gastroesophageal reflux disease) the latter of which I've had ongoing problems with as well. The sources I read on the subject, clearly distinguish asthmatic bronchitis from chronic bronchitis but both are considered diseases of COPD by some of them. Not a surprise, sense asthma itself is referred to as a form of COPD by many reputable medical sources as well. Still, the meaning I take from some of these articles, is that asthmatic bronchitis, actually has a better prognosis if properly treated than does chronic bronchitis, which in the majority of cases, is caused by long-term cigarette smoking.

Asthmatic bronchitis is not smoking-caused, although I'm sure this can be a contributing factor and it is often experienced in children. The med-sources I read on the condition also stated that the condition can be triggered in people, after their experiencing upper respiratory viruses and infections.

In some cases, antibiotics are used to get the condition under control but the general treatments for it, are the same as with typical asthma, including inhaled corticosteroid/glucocorticoid steroids and bronchodilator medications. It's my understanding that a good pulmonary doctor knows how to recognize the condition and to differentiate it from typical asthma. If you want to see information on the condition, use "asthmatic bronchitis" as a search term, which will yield you lots of information on the subject.

I hope my sharing what I generally learned about this condition was helpful! Blessings to all my fellow asthma patients!"

In Conclusion:

Many of us who are asthma patients, have ongoing problems, such as difficulty finding adequate doctors and getting proper treatment or even the correct diagnosis of our asthma types but we must remain diligent in getting adequate health care. Poorly treated asthma, can cause an undue worsening of asthmatic conditions and a progression toward lung damage. Self-education is also very important because this can give us additional hints on how to take care of ourselves, apart from the needed prescribed treatments by our doctors.

While asthma and related chronic respiratory disorders have no cures, we can remain inspired to achieve and maintain the best possible quality of life for ourselves, with the help of our doctors. While I realize there were a few negative aspects of asthma treatment discussed in this book, it is my hope that these will help patients to remain proactive in their cases, to avoid unnecessary negative experiences, regarding inadequate treatment and unqualified doctors.

I will add that there are wonderful doctors who treat asthmatic patients, who are passionate and certainly looking out for their patient's best interests. This scenario can be even better, when patients partner with their doctors, to the best of their ability, following their treatment-plans, as adequately as possible and reporting any significant symptom-changes to their doctors.

In closing, I would like to extend my sincere "Best Wishes" to my fellow asthma patients, who may read this book and it is my hope that you find helpful nuggets of information within the preceding pages.

-Jim Lowrance

About the Author:

I am a husband, father, grandfather and lifetime contract salesman, with experience in health writing that began in 2004. I completed theological studies with Liberty University in 1996. I formerly served as editor and forum moderator of Thyroid Health for a major multi-topic content site and as a general health writer for another, where I achieved Editor's Choice Awards for my articles on health subjects.

In 2003 I was diagnosed with hypothyroidism; "Hashimoto's thyroiditis" being the cause. This autoimmune form of thyroid disease that causes destruction of the thyroid gland resulted in my also developing "Chronic Fatigue Syndrome", due to a compromised immune system with severe co-morbid "Adrenal Fatigue". I also suffered severe anxiety symptoms, including panic attacks early into the onset of Hashimoto's thyroiditis (Hashitoxicosis). I was also diagnosed with peripheral neuropathy and thyroid myopathy, with co-morbid nutritional deficiencies. Additionally, I am a treated asthmatic patient, with GERD (Gastroesophageal reflux disease), as a major contributing factor to its development.

My eventual receiving of diagnoses was a difficult process with proper diagnostic testing not being ordered by the first doctors I sought treatment from. These types of issues were inspiration for me to become proactive in my own health care and to self-educate myself on these health disorders, which I have done extensively since 2003. I now enjoy sharing this information with other patients.